Introduction

After 38 years as a general practitioner in the Southern California area, I moved to the Northern California area. Soon after moving in 2010, patients began asking me about Medical Marijuana. Like most practitioners, my initial experience with medical cannabis was its use to stimulate appetite and weight gain in terminally ill cancer patients. Like many practitioners, I saw cannabis help these patients to eat and gain weight. Then I saw cannabis used to treat neuropathy. Neuropathy is very painful and difficult to treat. The cannabis not only helped the pain better than anything else, but improved the patient's appetite, sleep, and general wellbeing. It not only treated the resistant pain condition, but cannabis comforted the suffering patient better than any medicine I had seen before. Furthermore, this was accomplished without the distressing side effects of the powerful pharmaceuticals. As I saw more medical cannabis patients, they described to me condition after condition successfully treated with medical cannabis. Many diagnoses were what would be expected: anxiety, anorexia, and insomnia. But these were only a portion of the diagnoses. Migraine came up again and again. Some days I felt as if migraine patients were all that I saw. But then there was also Crohn's disease, irritable bowel syndrome, fibromyalgia, ADHD, post-traumatic stress disorder, Tourette's syndrome and multiple sclerosis.[1]

I saw 4 patients with titanium joints who told me that cannabis gave the most relief of the chronic pain from the artificial joint. And I heard again and again the story of how this person was strong, living a normal healthy life until that awful day of the "accident." Whether the trauma was in combat, at work, or in a car accident, they had a similar experience. Initially, they had intensive medical care-surgery, physical therapy, opiates, etc. At first the therapy was helpful. But then after time, the therapy had done what it could and then the medicines begin to make them sick. At some point, they would use medical cannabis for the residual symptoms of the injury, and discontinue the other medicines because of their side effects.

Two patients come to mind as poignant examples of the unique effectiveness of this medicine. One patient was a woman in her 50s who had delivered five children. She was a small woman approximately 5 foot tall and 100 pounds. All five of her babies were more than 9 pounds. Her perineum was terribly damaged from the childbirth injuries, so she had surgery that placed plastic mesh in her perineum and vagina. After the surgery, she began to experience constant incapacitating pain in her pelvis. She was no longer able to sleep.

Her son asked her what was wrong, and upon hearing that she had such pelvic pain, he proceeded to obtain cannabis leaf made into a liquid that she could bathe in. Initially, she would bathe three times a day. After a period of weeks, the pain receded. She now is able to sit comfortably without pain and no longer requires cannabis baths.

Another patient was a middle aged man with severe chronic paranoid schizophrenia who was morbidly obese. In talking with him about his cannabis therapy, he stated that he had lost 60 pounds on cannabis. When I was reluctant to believe him, he told me his story. He is a lifelong severely disabled paranoid schizophrenic. His antipsychotic medicines are so powerful that he does little more than sleep, lie on the couch and eat when he takes them. For six months, he tried to convince his psychotherapist to let him take cannabis. His psychiatrist finally relented. The patient stopped his powerful antipsychotic medicine during the day, and used cannabis during the day in place of the antipsychotic. He then told me "Now, instead of lying on the couch and eating all day, I can drive to the ocean and have some fish and chips." And then he lost 60 pounds.

Dedication

This book is dedicated to you, the medical cannabis patient. You are conscientious and meticulous in learning and using the cannabis medicine. You are some of the best patients I have had the privilege of treating during my long career. And I hope this book helps people realize that this country and the world would benefit from medical cannabis. This medicine is safe and effective. It is much more than a party drug. It will benefit many people.

Disclaimer

This book is not a medical prescription. Initiation of medical cannabis therapy or changes in your present therapy should only be done under close medical supervision of practitioners who are qualified in your specific illness and cannabis medical therapy.

Migraine, Menses, and Medical Marijuana

The association of the menstrual period and migraine is recorded by Hippocrates about 450 BC. He stated that "shivering, lassitude and heaviness of the head denotes the onset of menstruation." He was the first to describe the onset of the headache as a shining light followed by head pain that occupies the entire head.[2]

In 1666, Dutch physician Johannis van der Linden described a particularly severe case of one sided headache with nausea and vomiting associated with menstruation in the Marchioness of Brandenberg. [3]

Morris Fishbein,MD, editor of the Journal of the AMA stated in 1935"Some women find that their migraine attacks come with their period...[4]" And in 1942, Dr Fishbein stated " In this instance the patient may be given … fluidextract of cannabis three days before the onset of the menstrual period….The dose of the fluidextract of cannabis is five drops three times daily, increased daily by one drop until eleven drops, three times daily, are taken. Then the dosage is reduced by one drop daily until 5 drops are taken three times daily and so on."[5]

Why did the public spokesperson for the AMA state one year after cannabis had been removed from the US pharmacy that he recommends cannabis specifically for migraine triggered by menstruation?

We will begin our discussion of migraine and marijuana with some modern case histories. These case histories are from the writings of Dr Tod H Mikuriya(1933-2007). "Dr. Tod" was a psychiatrist known as the grandfather of medical cannabis. These case studies are from his professional papers, which are now kept at the National Institute of Health.[6]

Case study of modern migraine patient #1

Edie L., a thirty eight year old pert, intense, intelligent, articulate stock broker and former law student suffers from severe one-sided headaches that started when she was eleven years old. Aggravated by bacon, wines, monosodium glutamate, soy sauce, and complicated by severe menstrual cramping, she had been virtually house bound for weeks at a time. If the immobilizing pain, nausea, and depression from the attacks weren't bad enough, the side effects from conventional pharmacotherapy wrought further dysfunction.

Sedatives like phenobarbital and minor tranquilizers like Valium and Ativan left her sleepy and oversedated. Trips to the emergency room were frequent where Demerol (meperidine) and ergotamine (up to 3 injections in 24 hours) would bring the attack under control.

She had been to numerous specialists and underwent extensive workups including spinal taps, brain wave studies, xrays, allergy tests, and psychiatric interviews.

She made the observation that if she smoked marijuana just as the symptoms of an attack were starting that the attack could be kept at bay or stopped. She told this to several specialists who were treating her but this was either ignored or dismissed.

Because I could not prescribe marijuana Marinol was prescribed. Starting dropwise from puncturing a 10 milligram capsule using a method described by Dr. J. Russell Reynolds in 1890: "The dose should be given in minimum quantity, repeated in not less than four or six hours, and gradually increased by one drop every third or fourth day, until either relief is obtained, or the drug is proved, in such case, to be useless."

Actually, the adjustment of the dose came more easily. She found that her response to Marinol was not exquisitely sensitive and within several days she found that 10 milligrams two or three times a day was sufficient. The migraine attacks ceased. Subjectively, the Marinol did not cause sedation or immobility as with the other drugs but produced a feeling of well-being and relieved feelings of depression. The other medications worsened feelings of depression and immobility.

The expense of Marinol was, unfortunately prohibitive, causing her to have to resort to illicit cannabis of varying potency. Because of her continuing intermittently severe recurrent depression and premigraine anxiety, she has been unable to return to work. On follow-up four years later she has had "..only one meperidine trip to the emergency room in the past two years." She makes oral preparations using inexpensive Mexican marijuana. She complains of not being able to optimize the potency of her confections because of the varying potencies and small quantities she must prepare. She also must resort to smoking marijuana which is her route of least preference. Notwithstanding, the use of cannabis for the treatment of migraine headache and depression has proven to be better than any of the previous conventional drug treatments she has been prescribed.

Dr Mikuriya's Comments

Edie's case is not without precedent. A physician of a century ago would have prescribed cannabis in one of the many purified preparations that were available. Today, most physicians, including headache specialists, are unaware of this and or that Marinol is one of the active principles of cannabis.

Migraine Headache is a specific type of pain for which cannabis was first described to be useful by J. Russell Reynolds. After some thirty years clinical experience after this initial observation, he described "Migraine: very many victims have for years kept their sufferings in abeyance by taking hemp at the moment of threatening, or onset of the attack." In Osler's medical text it was the treatment of choice for migraine headache. The most recent (and last) mention of cannabis for the treatment of migraine was from Morris Fishbein, M.D., Editor of the Journal of the American Medical Association in 1942.

Case #2

Edie's mother, a 58 year old hospital ward clerk who has experienced migraine headaches with similar symptoms but less profoundly debilitating than those of her daughter. Likewise, she was treated with a gradually increasing dosage of Marinol with stabilization at a 10 mg daily dose (5 mg BID).Notwithstanding her undergoing stressful conditions on the job she experienced successful stopping of episodes in prodromal stage.

Left neck numbness, anorexia, water retention and left diplopia were reversed with normalization of gastric motility, diuresis, and peripheral vasodilation. She subjectively felt a relief of affectual pressure. She experienced no debilitating side effects as with other antimigraine agents and sedatives. Perceptually she described a "shift of vision"- slightly out of focus. This effect was transient.

Case #3

A 44 year old female teacher has a thirty year history of familial unilateral severe vascular headaches with antecedent visual scotomata. She switched to self-medication with marijuana after 9 years of meperidine/sedative treatments with their impairing effects.

Cases #4 & #5

Patient #3 taught her daughters ages 21 and 17 to self-medicate with marijuana with similar success in aborting migraine headaches in the prodromal phase with scotomata.

Case #6 is Dr Grinspoon's case study of a modern migraine patient and is very similar to Dr. Mikuriya's studies mentioned above.

Case # 6

"I first experienced a migraine in a classroom when I was 14. The sparkling, flickering affects, which were curious at first, consumed me so that I could not see the black board. I asked to be excused, let myself into the nurses' room and vomited for several hours until my mother came to get me.

After this happened several times, my mother took me to see my doctor, a close friend and neighbor who I saw very often because I had a lot of allergies. He and my mother agreed that the headaches were caused by the recent death of my baby sister, and he gave me nothing for the nausea and pain. Although headaches with some regularity, it wasn't until college that I was given the diagnosis of migraine and received medication. The college infirmary prescribed Ecotrin (coated aspirin), which helped somewhat with the headache but not the visual effects or the nausea. It also gave me tremendous heartburn.

One time the pain was so severe they gave me an injection of Demerol (a synthetic opioid). Which pretty completely wiped out the pain but left me very light headed. At times I took banana flavored syrup (probably codeine) which made me very sleepy.

I remembered it was difficult to make it through final exams because I was so light headed....

Several years later the migraines returned and my husband said he had read that marijuana was good for headaches. I was amazed. Two hits and a short rest completely warded off the nausea and headache. As soon as I noticed flickering visuals that forewarned me of an approaching migraine, I could take a little cannabis and a short nap and the migraine would not develop at all. I was usually ready to go back to work in a half hour. It gave me a feeling of tremendous power to finally be in control of my migraines.

In the 18 years that I began to use cannabis for the relief of migraines, I have been caught away from home with out my herb. Once I tried taking Tylenol and it helped a little with the pain but not at all with the nausea or the visual effects. Both of my older daughters, (now 17 and 21) also get occasional migraines, which appeared when they began to menstruate. Both get tremendous relief from cannabis herb. My mother suffers from severe headaches, but she has never used cannabis because it is illegal. She has a horrible time with the medication prescribed for her- nausea, constipation, high blood pressure. I often tell her that when marijuana is legal and she uses it for the first time and she realizes that she has suffered unnecessarily all these years, she is going to be really furious"!

Discussion by Dr Mikuriya
Hemp drugs (cannabis) were introduced to western medicine by O'Shaughnessy in 1839 and attained wide usage until the turn of the century. With the development of synthetic and semisynthetic analgesics, their use declined though maintaining mention in medical texts until removal from the formulary in 1940. Reclassified as a schedule I drug in 1970 alleged to having no medicinal redeeming importance, the synthetic THC created by government sponsored research contractors was downscheduled to schedule II in 1986, the same as non-combination opiates requiring triplicate prescription.

Definition of Migraine

True or classic migraine is a very specific group of symptoms. Even before the headache pain begins unusual symptoms can occur. Sparkling spots before the eyes, blindness in one eye, weakness of one side of the body, dizziness, trouble speaking, or thirst start just before the headache. Then the pain starts. The pain is usually in the same place every time. Nausea, vomiting, and sensitivity to light and sound often follow.

Common migraine is more frequent than classic migraine. It is a massive headache thru the entire head. Often nausea, vomiting, and sensitivity to light and sound occur.

Thirty-six million Americans suffer from migraine.

Cause

The brain in migraine sufferers is hyper excitable to a variety of stimuli. Migraine sufferers have a genetic defect in processing sensory stimuli such as light or sound. The cause of most true migraines is a genetic defect in a small number of nerves deep within the brain. All migraine genes so far identified increase neuronal excitability through a variety of mechanisms.

This defect translates normal stimuli like an average sun shining day, into an intense feeling of light, as if a powerful spotlight were located two inches before your eye. The normal stimulus is magnified to a level of intense pain. This processing error in the nervous system causes the nerves in the brain to fire too rapidly. Next the nerves fire off in intense waves that occur at 3-5 mm per/ second. These waves move thru the brain like a tsunami of electrons. These waves set off the visual effects (flashing lights, temporary blindness), nausea, and sensitivity to light and sound. These waves of electrical activity are followed by the pain in the head. After the wave of excessive firing of the neurons, they become burned out or depressed. This cycle of overstimulation followed by depression can go on for hours or days.

Treatment

There are more than ten different drugs for the treatment of migraine. Eight of them are only effective in the early stages of the headache. About two of every five migraine patients do not get adequate relief from the medicines for acute migraine. The medicines used for prevention of migraine are not very effective for many people. See Appendix A.

Of the ten medicines, the triptans (5HT1 agonists) are the most effective for migraine. But they can have very serious side effects and are expensive. Triptans do not prevent migraine. Opiates can be effective, but have many serious side effects, and can easily lead to overdose and/or addiction.

As Dr Joel Saper, director of the Michigan Headache and Neurological Institute, a treatment and research center in Ann Arbor, Michigan says, "There is no universally effective therapy. What might be a miracle drug for one person could be a dud for another."

One fact agreed upon by all experts is that if the migraine headache can be treated quickly and immediately after the onset of the attack, many medicines can be effective in stopping the headache.

My own professional experience with thousands of migraine sufferers in the primary care setting has demonstrated that somewhere between 10-40% of patients will not be completely relieved by any or all of the medicines above. Many times the side effects are too toxic for the patient. A small percentage (5-10%) never gets relief with any of the above medications.

History of Cannabis for Migraines

There is a long history of cannabis treating and preventing migraine. The first member of western culture to study cannabis was William O'Shaughnessy in 1839. He did not prescribe cannabis for migraine, but following his introduction of cannabis to western culture, numerous practitioners began prescribing cannabis for migraines. In appendix B there are 30 examples of practitioners who recommended cannabis for the treatment of migraine in the 19th and 20th centuries.

In 1913 Sir William Osler stated in his classic medical text book, "Principles and Practice of Medicine (8th edition)",

"Cannabis is probably the best medicine for migraine."

Also Dr. Ringer in 1892 wrote,

""No single drug have I found so useful in Migraine." He (Ringer) thinks it acts well in all forms, but seems most useful in preventing rather than arresting."

The best description of the effectiveness of Cannabis in treating migraine comes from Dr HA Hare,

"Tincture or extract of cannabis were our best remedies in the treatment of migraine….In true migraine with hemianopsia, this treatment is often most effectual in aborting the attack. The prevention of attacks is to be attained by the use of smaller amounts of cannabis during the intervals."

Dr Hare describes a true or classical migraine headache attack. We know this because the headache is associated with hemianopsia, which is the loss of vision of half of one or both eyes at the same time.

This finding is characteristic of classical migraine. This means that cannabis "is often most effectual in aborting the attack" of classical migraine. And he also tells us "prevention of attacks is to be attained by the use of smaller amounts of cannabis during the intervals".

Mattison, Green, and Ringer also stated that cannabis was preventive as well as able to "abort" the acute headache. These are five medical experts who state that cannabis prevents migraine. Twenty other experts who write that cannabis is effective in treating acute migraine are listed in Appendix B. This was the state of the art of medicine when Dr Hare wrote his statement above in 1922.

In the 20th century cannabis was removed from the US Pharmacopeia in 1942. Therefore present day doctors know very little about medical cannabis.

Because of the prohibition of medical cannabis in the US, there are only two 20th century studies on medical cannabis for chronic headache sufferers. In one study 3 chronic headache sufferers found relief through medical cannabis. (Noyes and Barton,1974). Another study showed 3 headache sufferers who stopped their long term medical cannabis treatment for migraine suffered return of their headaches after stopping cannabis. (El Mallakh,1987)

Psychiatrist Tod Mikuriya, MD reported in his professional papers five cases of classic migraine successfully treated by medical cannabis. In three cases, consisting of a mother and her two daughters, all three suffered migraine with hemianopsia that was aborted by cannabis.

So we see Dr Hare in 1891 and Dr Mikuriya in 1991 describing migraine with hemianopsia aborted by cannabis.

In a recent study (Sarchielli, 2007) of severe migraine sufferers, samples of the cerebral spinal fluid were found to be low in the naturally occurring endocannabinoids, AEA and 2AG. This means that the fluid that bathes the brain in severe headache sufferers is low in endocannabinoids. This is evidence of an endocannabinoids deficiency state that could cause migraine headache.

Recent Clinical Experience

Because California allows medical cannabis for patients I have seen several hundred patients with migraine successfully treated with cannabis. Although this is a small number of patients it is enough to establish that to a significant number of migraine sufferers, their migraines are treated and controlled with cannabis. Several medical cannabis doctors are quoted in O'Shaughnessy magazine as stating that 10% of their consultations are for migraine. This finding may be evidence that medical cannabis can relieve that 5-10% of resistant migraine sufferers whose pain is not relieved by the other migraines medications now available.

Conclusion

This describes our present day situation in which there is a large amount of evidence from doctors who had experience with the drug from about 1840 to the 1930's. Over 20 authorities from that time period state that cannabis treats and prevents migraines. The two studies available to us since cannabis prohibition are consistent with cannabis treating migraine. Modern medical research shows that severe sufferers of migraines have cerebral spinal fluid bathing the brain that is low in endocannabinoids. And the experience of medical cannabis doctors, including myself, is that cannabis not only treats the acute migraine but also prevents recurring migraines. This experience of modern day use of medical cannabis consultants is consistent with the experience of the physicians of the past who were able to prescribe cannabis and is totally consistent with migraine being caused by an endocannabinoid deficiency state in the central nervous system.

How to Treat and Prevent Migraine with Medical Cannabis

"Tincture or extract of cannabis were our best remedies in the treatment of migraine….In true migraine with hemianopsia, this treatment is often most effectual in aborting the attack. **The prevention of attacks is to be attained by the use of smaller amounts of cannabis during the intervals"**

Hare, Hobart Amory, MD, *Practical Therapeutics*, Phil, Pa, 1922

Hare, 1887 "Within a few years this drug has become particularly prominent in connection with its use in migraine… **I have certainly seen very severe and intractable cases of migraine successfully treated by this remedy, not only in regard to the attack itself, but by acting as a prophylactic. If the attacks are frequent then the remedy should be used constantly in small doses, in such a way that the patient is not conscious of any influence of the drug, and about 1/8 of a grain of the solid extract may be taken night and morning, or, if this produces any tendency to sleep, the whole may be taken at night. At the beginning and during the attack it should be freely administered until either the pain is diminished or very marked symptoms of its physiologic action assert**
themselves.

Cases of migraine treated in this way, when the disease does not depend on any distinct organic lesion, are in large proportion of instances either entirely cured or greatly benefited, the attacks, even when they recur being considerably farther apart." Hare, MD, Hobart Amory, *Clinical and physiological notes on the action of cannabis Indica*, The Therapeutic Gazette, vol. II,1887, pp. 225-228

As Dr. Hare states above, based on his more than 35 years of experience with medical cannabis with migraine, medical cannabis is effective both in the acute migraine setting as well as in chronic, frequent migraine. As stated in the previous chapter on migraine, three other authors with long-term experience in migraine and medical cannabis write that medical cannabis is curative for migraine.[7]

Treatment of Acute Migraine

"At the beginning and during the attack it should be freely administered until either the pain is diminished or very marked symptoms of its physiologic action assert themselves."(Hare)

All authorities agree that all treatment modalities are most effective when the treatment of the acute migraine is started as soon as possible after the beginning of the symptoms. This means it is best to initiate treatment at the first sign of aura.

Treatment should start with inhaled medical cannabis. The effect of cannabis is very rapid when inhaled. The inhaled THC goes immediately into the arterial circulation and quickly reaches the brain. Because the THC is lipid soluble, the THC molecule moves quickly through the blood brain barrier. The blood brain barrier slows down the water soluble neurotransmitters, such as adrenaline and opiates, from passing through into the brain. But because THC is a small lipid molecule, it has been described as "flying" quickly through the blood brain barrier and quickly exerting its central nervous affects. This rapid inhalation of the fat-soluble THC through the lungs, directly into the bloodstream, and quickly through the blood brain barrier is the physiologic reason why THC has such a quick onset of action.

This rapid onset of action, which bypasses the gastrointestinal tract, is very close to being as rapid in onset as intravenous medications. In migraine, the fastest route of the most effective treatment is subcutaneous sumatriptan. I have had several patients tell me that inhaled cannabis was even better for the treatment of migraine than subcutaneous sumatriptan. One individual related to me that for many years he never left the house without a syringe with injectable sumatriptan. He then reported to me that after using cannabis on a regular basis, he no longer suffered migraine and stopped carrying his injectable sumatriptan.

After beginning inhaled cannabis therapy as soon as possible after the onset of symptoms, the medicine is inhaled frequently in small to medium doses until the pain is felt to decrease. The goal is to push the initial dose of inhaled cannabis until the pain is gone or negative side effects require the patient to decrease the medicine. If negative side effects require that the medicine be decreased in amount, one need only wait approximately 15 to 30 minutes before the negative side effects diminish. Then the medicine could be reinstituted with a smaller dose at frequent intervals.

Treatment of Chronic Migraine

This treatment method of quickly initiating inhaled cannabis therapy will control the pain of migraine in most cases. But it soon becomes cumbersome to smoke many times in a day. A much easier method of cannabis ingestion is an oral preparation. The standard dose of THC that is required each day to keep away the migraines with inhaled cannabis is converted to an equivalent daily edible THC dose. This dose is worked out individually for each patient.

The daily edible THC dose is divided into two equal parts. The first dose is given in the morning. The second dose is given in the evening before bed. The inhaled THC medicine is always available. If there is a breakthrough of the migraine pain, the inhaled cannabis is once again used in the manner stated above. Namely, that the inhaled THC medication is begun immediately on noticing the breakout of the pain. The inhaled medication is used frequently and in small doses. Inhaling medicine every 30 to 60 minutes is common during this kind of problem. When pain control is achieved, then the inhaled cannabis medication is stopped. An increase in the elixir dose is started, using the smallest possible increments. The inhaled cannabis is always available to augment the edible cannabis. Whenever possible, the patient tries to choose the smallest dose effective to stop the pain, whether the route of administration is oral or inhaled cannabis. Sometimes the daily edible dose causes too much sedation when divided into two equal doses. In that case, a smaller dose could be given in the morning. For instance, the dose could be divided into one part in the morning and three parts in the evening. And if this decrease in the daytime dose is not satisfactory, then the entire daily edible dose of cannabis could be given in the evening just before bed.

Menses

Now that we have studied migraine and cannabis, let us move on to the discomfort and pain caused by the menstrual period. Dr Grinspoon describes a case of a modern woman with difficult, painful periods.

Modern Case Study

This this is the testimony of Judy F, who in 1993 was a 35-year-old administrative assistant to a Wall Street broker:

"I have used marijuana for many years to alleviate the symptoms of premenstrual syndrome-bloating, headaches, mood swings, and anxiety. I also use it to relieve cramping and fatigue during the menstrual cycle itself. I have tried conventional medicines such as aspirin, acetaminophen, and ibuprofen. Only ibuprofen has any effect; it illuminates cramping: but only in a triple dose that causes increased bloating, drowsiness, and constipation. When I start to experience the confusion, anger, and hypersensitivity that signal the onset of a premenstrual mood swing, smoking a joint is the one remedy that works immediately to soothe my nerves. It is as if my whole system has been slowed to put everything in order. My thought processes are less jumbled; I reacted less impulsively and become more rational. If I smoke half a joint at night, I sleep better. My husband of six years has attested to these effects many times.

For these last five years I have worked in a fast-paced and tense environment that requires me to keep a clear head and make important decisions. On a normal day smoking pot might be detrimental to my performance, but when I am premenstrual, it becomes necessary if I am to function at my usual capacity. I'll go outside and take a few hits off a joint, and by the time I return, I feel much more in control. I'm able to organize my work and think each task through. I usually smoke at two hour intervals. My employer and some of my coworkers are aware of the situation, and they support me fully, even though they do not smoke marijuana themselves. I recently gave a woman at my workplace, a joint during her menstrual period, and she came in the next morning raving about how it eased her cramps and decreased her anxiety."

Many of the 19th and 20th century authors mentioned above in the Migraine section used cannabis for treatment of menstrual problems. In the 1800-1900's, menstrual problems would have included both premenstrual and menstrual problems and pains. In other words the doctors of that day would have used medical cannabis for what we call today premenstrual dysphoric disorder (PMDD and PMS) and painful periods.

Also practitioners of that day as well as today knew that many women suffered migraines before their periods came. For some women, the only time they experience migraine is immediately before their period. This is consistent with a link between the menstrual period and the migraine. Appendix B has seven examples of practitioners during the 1840-1930 time period who stated that cannabis is effective in treating painful periods.

As Les Grinspoon, MD writes, "cannabis was commonly used in the 19th century for the symptoms associated with the menstrual cycle."

J R Reynolds, Queen Victoria's physician, prescribed it for her for both premenstrual symptoms and menstrual cramps. During the reign of Queen Victoria the British Empire was very powerful. Subjects of the crown in India were producing the highest quality of cannabis for the Queen. Her doctor was one of the best doctors in the entire Empire. The best of medical cannabis and the best of medical care were able to control her menstrual symptoms without interfering in her many public duties.

The effect of THC on painful periods is reinforced by the recent discovery that CB2 receptors are found in the uterus.

Appendix A

Partial List of Treatments for Migraine

Drug	Side Effects	Effect	
Ergot	Aggravates HTN and heart disease	Moderately Effective	
Opiates	Constipation, confusion, addiction, death	Effective	
Triptans-now includes digital electronic skin patch	Can't be used in presence of heart disease, Chest pain	Effective	Very expensive and usually allowed no more than 4-6 doses/month
Beta Blockers	Sedation, fatigue	Not very effective	
Calcium channel blockers		Not very effective	
Aspirin/NSAID	Stomach upset	Moderately effective	
Chlorpromazine Thorazine	Very sedating	Moderately Effective	Only effective in acute setting
Barbiturates	Addictive, sedating, can	Not very effective	Overdose can be fatal

	easily overdose		
Cortisone	Multiple dangerous side effects	Not very effective	
Magnesium IV	Used only in ER	Effective Doesn't prevent	
Tricyclic, SNRI Antidepressant	Many side effects	Somewhat effective	Best for prevention
Botox Injections		Unknown	Only FDA appoved treatment for migraine
Occipital Nerve Stimulation		Unknown	
Transcranial Direct Current stimulation (of occiput)		Unknown	
Meditation (Mindfulness)		Unknown	

Appendix B

Authorities who state that cannabis treats Migraine headaches

1 Osler, MD William, "Concerning migraine headache, Osler stated in his text: Cannabis Indica is probably the most satisfactory remedy."
Osler, W., and McCrae, T.: Principles and Practice of medicine, 8th edition,

D. Appleton and Company. New York, 1916 p. 1089. *Mikuriya, Tod, Marijuana: Medical Papers Volume I*, pg. xviii

2 "Tincture or extract of cannabis were our best remedies in the treatment of migraine….In true migraine with hemianopsia, this treatment is often most effectual in aborting the attack. The prevention of attacks is to be attained by the use of smaller amounts of cannabis during the intervals"

Hare, HA, MD, Practical Therapeutics, Phil, Pa, 1922; pg. 181 ibid pg. 114

3 Ringer says: "No single drug have I found so useful in Migraine." He thinks it acts well in all forms, but seems it most useful in preventing rather than arresting, Mattison, MD, JB: Cannabis Indica as an anodyne and hypnotic; the St. Louis Medical and Surgical Journal, volume LVI, no. 5, November 1891, pages 265-271. *Mikuriya, Vol I pg. 152*

4 "Seguin, in 1877, commended it highly," Seguin, Dr. EC; Mattison ibid, pg.

152

5 "Sinkler, in a paper on migraine, gives first place to cannabis, and thinks it of more value in this form than any other" Sinkler, Dr. W; Mattison,   (ibid, pg. 153)

6 "Richard Green, who first commended it in this complaint, thinks it not only relieves, but cures; in nearly all cases giving lasting relief." Mattison, ibid. pg. 153

7 Dr. Suckling, in the British Medical Journal, July 4, 1891. "Dr. Suckling, Professor of medicine, Queens College, Birmingham writes:" I have during the last few years been accustomed to prescribe Indian hemp in many conditions, and this drug seems to me to deserve a better repute than it has obtained…. In migraine, the drug is of great value; a pill containing one half grain of the extract … often immediately checks an attack, and if the pill be given twice a day continuously, the severity of frequency of the attacks are often much diminished. I have met with patients who have been incapacitated for work from the frequency of the attacks, and who have been enabled by the use of Indian hemp to resume their employment." Mattison, Ibid, page 153

8 "Anstie commends it in migraine…..From ¼ to1/2 grain of good extract of cannabis….is an excellent remedy in migraine of the young." Mattison ibid,

9 "Russell Reynolds, MD thinks that in migraine…...it is by far the best of drugs." Mattison;   ibid, pg. 153

10"Donavan and Fuller claim it of value in migraine," Mattison ibid pg. 154

11 Mattison; "I close this paper by again asking attention to the need of giving hemp in migraine. Were its use limited to this alone, its worth, direct, and in direct, would be greater than most imagine. Bear in mind the bane of American women is headache. Recollect that hemp eases pain without disturbing stomach and secretions so often as opium, and that competent men think it not only calmative, but curative. ... My experience warrants this statement: cannabis Indica is, often, a safe and successful anodyne and hypnotic." Ibid, pg. 156-157

12 Hare, 1887 "Within a few years this drug has become particularly prominent in connection with its use in migraine… I have certainly seen very severe and intractable cases of migraine successfully treated by this remedy, not only in regard to the attack itself, but by acting as a prophylactic. If the attacks are frequent then the remedy should be use constantly in small doses, in such a way that the patient is not conscious of any influence of the drug, and about 1/8 of a grain of the solid extract may be taken night and morning, or, if this produces any tendency to sleep, the whole may be taken at night. At the beginning and during the attack it should be freely administered until either the pain is diminished or very marked symptoms of its physiologic action assert themselves. Cases of migraine treated in this way, when the disease does not depend on any distinct organic lesion, are in large proportion of instances either entirely cured or greatly benefited, the attacks, even when they recur being considerably farther apart." Hare, Hobart Amory, Clinical and physiological notes on the action of cannabis Indica, The Therapeutic Gazette, vol. II,1887, pp. 225-228 ibid, pg. 293-295

13 Reynolds, R; "Migraine: Very many victims of this malady have for years kept their suffering in ….. By taking hemp at the moment of threatening, or onset of their attack", Therapeutical Uses, and Toxic Effects of Cannabis Indica, Lancet, volume 1, March 22, 1890, pp. 637-638. ibid, pg. 147

14 Remington, JP; "Cannabis is used in medicine to relieve pain….For its

analgesic action it is used especially in pains of neuralgic origin, such as migraine." 'The Dispensatory of the USA' 1914 ibid, pg. 343

15 "Reynolds, in 1890, summed up 30 years of clinical experience using cannabis, finding it useful and valuable in treating… migraine headache." Reynolds, R; Therapeutical Uses, and Toxic Effects of Cannabis Indica, Lancet, volume 1, March 22, 1890, pp. 637-638. ibid, pg. xvii

17 Noyes and Baram(1974) reported on 5 patients who used cannabis to treat painful conditions, of whom 3 had chronic headaches. All three subjects reported relief that was comparable or superior to Ergotamine Tartrate and Aspirin.
Holland, pg. 334

19 El Mallakh (1987) presented three cases in which abrupt cessation of frequent, prolonged daily marijuana smoking resulted in severe migraine attacks, Holland, pg. 334

20 Farlow considered cannabis useful in "nervous headache." McKenzie said that it is the valued remedy he has met with in the treatment of persistent headache. Marshall does not consider that cannabis is generally useful but says however that it appears to be useful in a headache of a dull and continuance character.
    Walton et al, Marijuana: America's new drug problem (JB Lippincott, 1938), ibid pg. 162

21 "Regarding migraine Stevens says that cannabis Indica is sometimes useful" Walton et al, ibid, pg. 162

22 "Osler and McCrae have said that for migraine that cannabis indica is the most satisfactory remedy. However in the latest edition of this text is only suggested that "a prolonged course of cannabis Indica may be tried." Solis-Cohen and Githens consider that Cannabis is of great service in certain cases of migraine" Walton et al, …ibid, pg. 162

23 "Fantus recently recommended its use in migraine… Walton et AL, Ibid,

pg.162
24 "N.F. McConnell, Bastedo, Hare, Lewis, and Bragman have also

favorably mentioned its use in migraine." Walton, RP, Marijuana: America's new drug problem (JB Lippincott, 1938), pp. 151-157. ibid page 163

25 Chronic Migraine Headache: five cases successfully treated with Marinol and/or illicit cannabis.
Tod H. Mikuriya, M.D., Schaffer Library of Drug Policy,
www.druglibrary.org

Case 1
A thirty eight year old white female stock broker supervisor with a twenty-six year history of unilateral vascular headaches escalating to generalized headache with tension headache overlay. The severity and frequency of episodes responded only to parenteral dihydroergotamine, meperidine, and trimethobenzamide HCl with sedation and further immobilization.

Marinol (delta 1-9 tetrahydrocannabinol dissolved in sesame oil) was begun with gradual upward titration dropwise to avoid undesirable mental side effects. She experienced a significant decrease in the frequency of attacks except when she ran out of medication.

She tolerated 40 mg daily (10 mg QID) without side effects but experienced an attack after running out of the THC capsules. Because of financial straits secondary to her disability status and the high expense of Marinol she has partially substituted illicitly obtained marijuana which she has ingested orally with similar relief.

Over the past four years she has maintained better control over the attacks with only one trip to the emergency room for a meperidine treatment in the past two years. She continues to utilize illicit cannabis because of the high cost of Marinol but has difficulty with irregular dosage with either too little or too much.

Case 3
It would appear that further clinical trial of both Marinol and cannabis for the treatment of migraine headache would be desirable.
References

Fishbein, M Queries and Minor Notes: Migraine Associated With Menstruation JAMA Vol 120:4 Sept 26, 1942 p 326

Grinspoon L and Baklar; Marijuana Forbidden Medicine

Mackenzie, S.; Indian hemp in persistent headache. JAMA 1887 9:732.

O'Shaughnessy, W.B.: On the preparations of the Indian Hemp or gunjah; their effects on the animal system in health and their utility in the treatment of tetanus and other convulsive diseases. Trans. Med. and Phys. Soc., Bengal, 1838-40; 71-102, 421-461.

Osler, W., and McCrae: Principles and Practice of Medicine. 8th ed., D. Appleton & Co., New York, 1916, p. 1809

Reynolds, JR: On Some Therapeutical Uses of Indian Hemp. Arch Med London 1859 Vol 2 154 - 160

Reynolds, JR: Therapeutical uses and toxic effects of cannabis indica. Lancet 1890 1; March 22: 637-638

Solis-Cohen, S. and Githens, T.S.: Pharmacotherapeutics, Materia Medica and Drug Action. D. Appleton and Co. New York, 1928.

Volfe, Z, Dvilansky, A, Nathan, I, Cannabinoids block release of serotonin from platelets induced by plasma from migraine patients. Int. J Clin Pharmacol. Res, 1985; 5(4): 243-6
September 12, 1991, Berkeley, CA

Appendix C

Authorities who state that cannabis treats Dysmenorrhea

1 "Ringer asserts it sometimes signally useful in dysmenorrhea." Mattison et al, ibid, pg. 154

2. "West commends it (cannabis) here (for dysmenorrhea)." Mattison et al, ibid, pg. 154

3. "Potter states that its anodyne (pain relieving) power is marked in....dysmenorrhea." Mattison et al, Potter, ibid, pg. 154

4. "Some have been particularly enthusiastic regarding the value of cannabis

in dysmenorrhea." Walton, RP, Marijuana: America's new drug problem (JB Lippincott, 1938), ibid pg. 164

5. "Reynolds, in 1890, summed up thirty years of his clinical experience using cannabis, finding it valuable in treating dysmenorrhea." Therapeutical uses, and toxic effects of cannabis Indica, Lancet, volume 1, March 22, 1890, pp. 637-638, ibid, pg. xvii

6. Dr. JP Willis of Royalston, " I have used the Indica Hemp for some time
dysmenorrhea." McMeens, RR, Report of the Ohio State Medical Committee on Cannabis Indica, transactions of the 15th Annual Meeting of the Ohio State Medical Society at Ohio White sulfur Springs, June 12-14, 1860, pp. 75-100. Ibid 117.

7. West, "Dr. West says the hemp is recommended in dysmenorrhea; "McMeens, et al ibid, pg. 124.

BIBLIOGRAPHY

Center for Medicinal Cannabis Research, www.cmcr.ucsd.edu

Epocrates.com, Migraine. Last accessed August 2013

Gerdeman and Lovinger, CB1 Cannabinoid Receptor Inhibits Synaptic Release of Glutamate in Rat Dorsal Striatum, Journal of Neurophysiology, Jan 2001, vol 85, no 1, 468-471

Grinspoon, MD L; Marihuana: the Forbidden Medicine, 1997, Yale University Press, New Haven,

Holland Julie; The Pot Book, 2010, Park Street Press, Rochester, VT

International Association for Cannabinoid Medicines, www.cannabis-med.org

Migraines Force Sufferers to Do Their Homework , NY Times, 1/29/2010

Mikuriya, Tod; Marijuana Medical Papers 1839-1972, Vol 1; 2007, Symposium Publishing, Nevada City, CA

Russo, Ethan,*Cannabis* the Migraine Treatment The Once and Future prescription?,Pain(1998), 3-8

Sarchielli, P et al, Endocannabinoids in chronic migraine: CSF findings suggest a system failure, Neuropsyhopharmacology, 2007 Jun; 32(6); 1432 (Pubmed)

Fishbein, M Queries and Minor Notes: Migraine Associated With Menstruation JAMA Vol 120:4 Sept 26, 1942 p 326

Chapter Two
The Science of Cannabis

Understanding of the chemistry of cannabis entered western culture with the

1839 work of

WB O'Shaughnessy, MD. A professor of medicine and surgery at Calcutta

medical school,

Dr. O'Shaughnessy became familiar with cannabis while in India. He made

studies on the effects of cannabis on animals and humans. Cannabis from the

Indian subcontinent was then introduced to Europe at the time of his return.

Because of the difficult chemistry of the compounds contained in cannabis,

mainly its fat soluble nature, it took many years to work out the structure.

The compound was not isolated until 1945. In 1964, Dr. Raphael Mechoulam of Hebrew University, determined the structure of the chemical compound that was the psychoactive part of the cannabis plant. That chemical is delta-9 tetrahydrocannabinol.

Figure 1 Delta-9 tetrahydrocannabinol

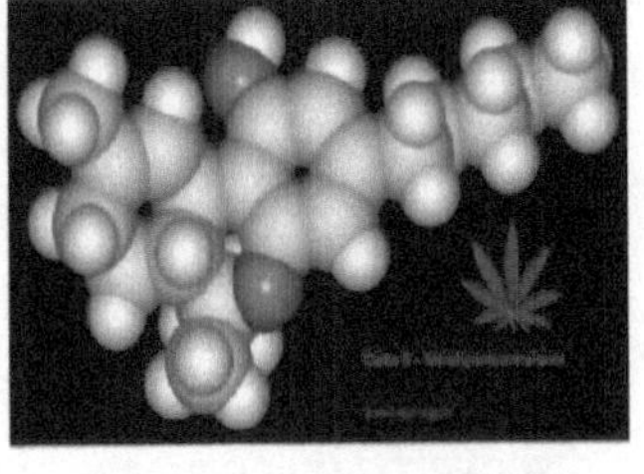

Even though the structure of the chemical compound was worked out, the action of THC was unknown. Up until 1988, THC was thought to disrupt the lipid portion of the cell membrane in some as yet unknown way.

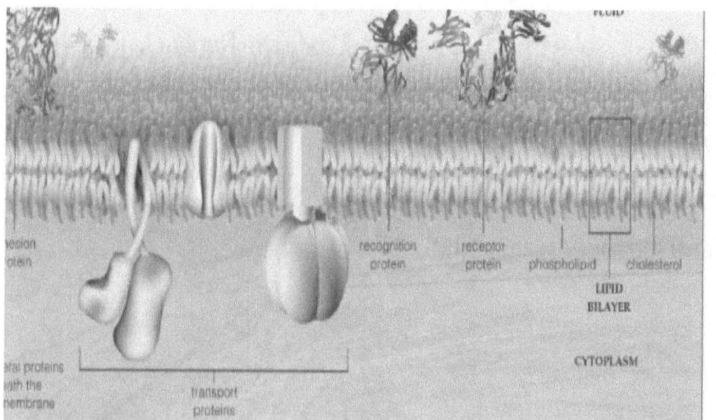

Figure 2 Cell membrane showing lipid bilayer. THC was thought to disrupt this like an anesthetic (dope). But we now know THC acts through a unique G receptor

This general cell membrane perturbation theory is how anesthetics such as ether and nitrous oxide are thought to work. Anesthetics disrupt the cell membrane in general, sort of beating up the cell membrane until the cell can't function at all.

However in 1988 it was discovered that cannabis worked through a cell membrane receptor called the G protein-coupled receptor. The fact that cannabis works through a G receptor means that the cannabinoids are part of our genes. Cannabis is not "dope", beating up on the cell membrane until the cell can't function. It is a unique key that fits a genetically determined lock, which is also unique. That unique lock is the cannabinoid G receptor. That key is the cannabinoid molecule, whether made by the body or ingested from outside the body.

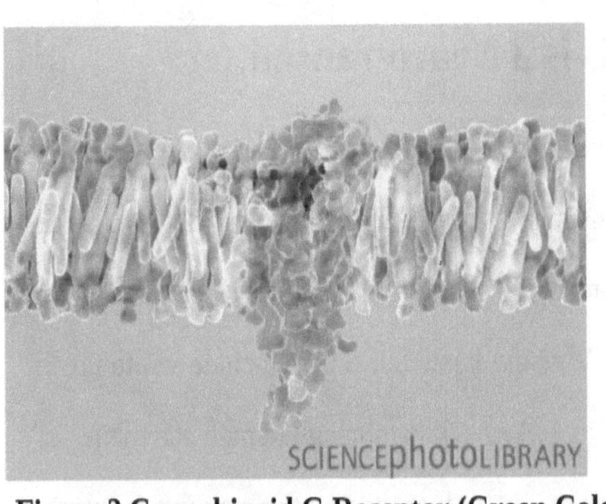

Figure 2 Cannabinoid G Receptor (Green Colored) The receptor is seen as a unique protein in the middle of the lipid bilayer.

This cannabis G receptor was first found inside the central nervous system. Since the human body has receptors to this chemical, Dr Mechoulam reasoned that there must be natural compounds produced by the human body to fit into the cannabis G receptors. Indeed, he found in 1992 the human produced natural cannabinoids (AEA &2-AG)[8] that correspond with the THC molecule from cannabis.

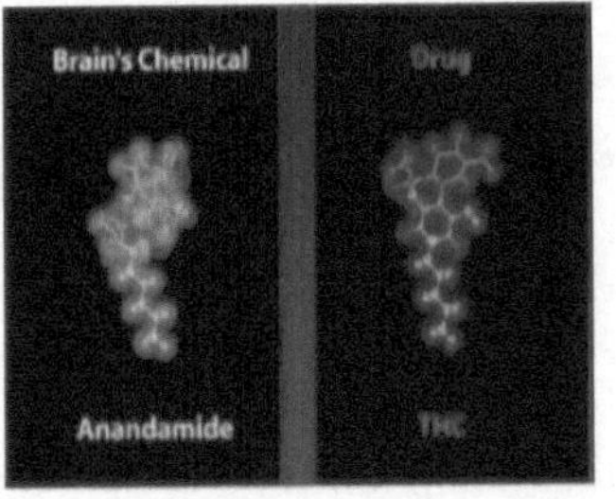

Figure 5 This photograph comapares the natural Endocannabinoid Anandamide (Left) with the Cannabis plant Exocannabinoid THC(Right)

Cannabis is a Neurotransmitter

Because endocannabinoids have their own unique G receptor, they are human neurotransmitters. Neurotransmitters are chemicals that flow between nerve cells to send a signal from one nerve cell (neuron) to another. There are more than 100 neurotransmitters. We only know 50. These include serotonin, opiate, adrenalin, noradrenalin, GABA, dopamine, glutamine and many others. The neurotransmitter acts as key that fits into the lock(G Receptor) of the pre-synaptic neuron. The effect of the key in the lock depends on what cell the G Receptor is located on. The cannabinoid receptors are located in most cells of the body.

This concept is illustrated in the figure below.

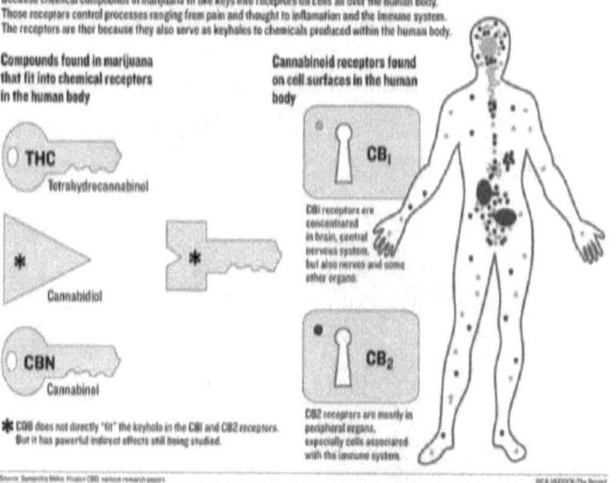

Please note that many other compounds other than the three listed in the above chart are present in the cannabis plant. A partial list is found illustrated in the chart below:

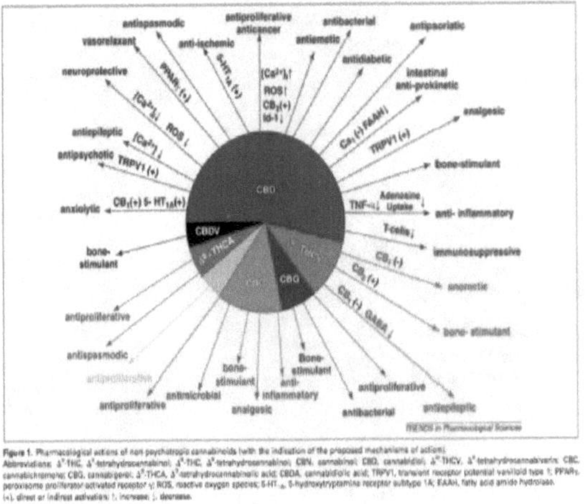

Figure 1. Pharmacological actions of non-psychotropic cannabinoids (with the indication of the proposed mechanisms of action). Abbreviations: Δ^9-THC, Δ^9-tetrahydrocannabinol; Δ^8-THC, Δ^8-tetrahydrocannabinol; CBN, cannabinol; CBD, cannabidiol; Δ^9-THCV, Δ^9-tetrahydrocannabivarin; CBC, cannabichromene; CBG, cannabigerol; Δ^9-THCA, Δ^9-tetrahydrocannabinolic acid; CBDA, cannabidiolic acid; TRPV1, transient receptor potential vanilloid type 1; PPARγ, peroxisome proliferator activated receptor γ; ROS, reactive oxygen species; 5-HT$_{1A}$, 5-hydroxytryptamine receptor subtype 1A; FAAH, fatty acid amide hydrolase. (+), direct or indirect activation; ↑, increase; ↓, decrease.

The diagram below shows the different parts of a nerve cell. The electricity that flows thru the neuron enters the neuron thru the dendrites, then down the axon to the end of the neuron where the terminal branches touch the next neuron.

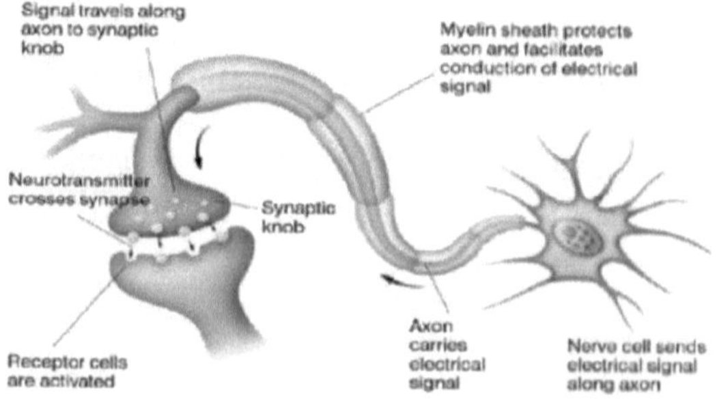

Figure 5   The Neuron(Nerve Cell)

The next figure shows how the neurons touch each other, an area called the synapse.

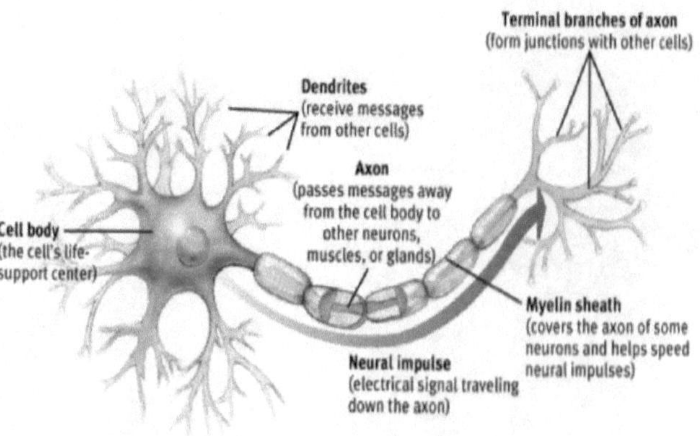

Figure 6 Neuron(Nerve Cell) Viewed from the Synapse

The diagram below magnifies the area where two nerve cells (neurons) come together, the synapse. The space between the two neurons is called the synaptic cleft.

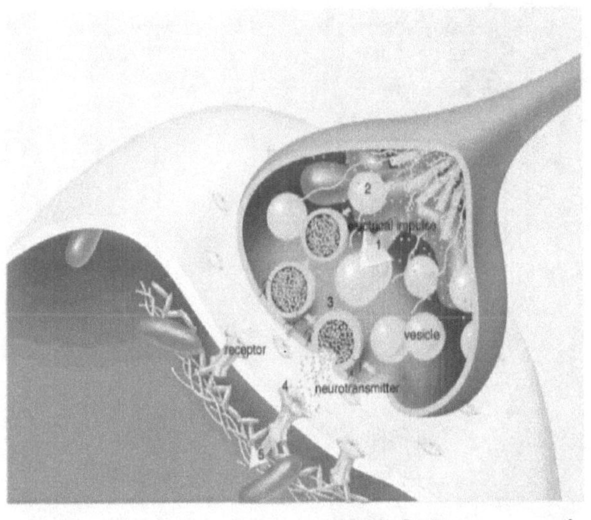

Figure 7 Nerve Synapse (Pink Presynaptic-Blue Postsynaptic)
The pink (presynaptic) nerve brings a signal to the blue (postsynaptic) neuron. The order of events is: (1) The yellow arrow shows the electrical impulse moving down toward the end of the neuron. (2) The green spheres are vesicles, which are containers filled with a neurotransmitter. The vesicle moves to the end of the neuron. (3) The vesicle empties all of its neurotransmitter into the cleft, or space between the neurons, (4) The neurotransmitter travels across the cleft between the neurons and is absorbed into the postsynaptic cell by a unique receptor,(5)After the neurotransmitter is absorbed by the receptor, it causes chemical reactions inside the postsynaptic neuron.

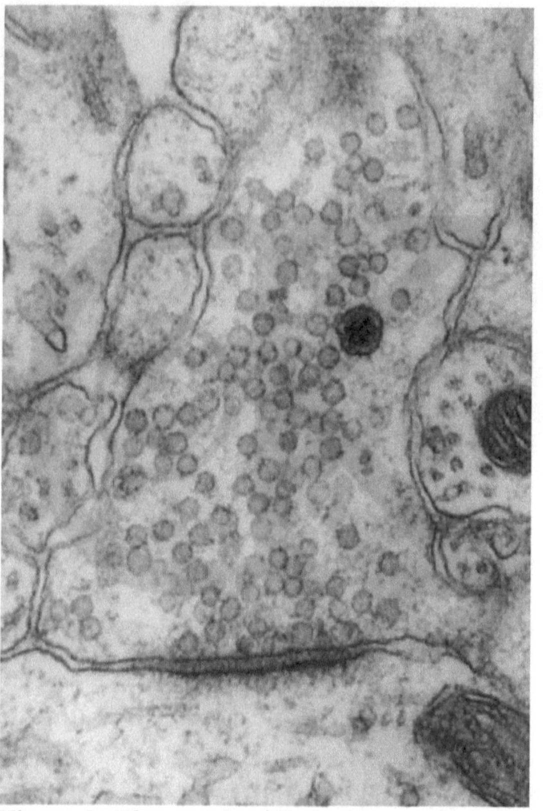

Figure 8   The vesicles filled with water soluble neurotransmitters (purple spheres above) occupy the end of the presynaptic neuron, spill over into the synaptic cleft, fill the cleft with neurotransmitter, which then penetrates into the post-synaptic cell.

Cannabinoids are reverse neurotransmitters

In 2003, the ground breaking scientific discovery that the endocannabinoids are reverse neurotransmitters or retrograde messengers was made.[9] The illustration above (Fig 7) shows the classic ante grade (downstream) flow of signal. The electrical signal causes the vesicles (containing chemical neurotransmitter) to move to the space (cleft) between the nerve cells, where the neurotransmitter is released from the presynaptic cell to the postsynaptic cell. The neurotransmitter travels across the cleft, where it is absorbed by the post synaptic neuron. All other neurotransmitters flow only one direction, "downstream" from the pre synaptic neuron to the postsynaptic neuron. And all other neurotransmitters are water-soluble molecules that are gathered into containers called vesicles that accumulate relatively large amounts of neurotransmitter molecules. These vesicles travel down the neuron to the presynaptic part of the neuron. When the vesicles reach the end of the neuron, they merge with the cell membrane and release large amounts of water soluble neurotransmitters into the presynaptic cleft at the same time. (See Fig. 9).

The water-soluble ante grade neurotransmitters can be produced far away from the neuron to be affected. For example, when a person is scared, the adrenal glands secrete adrenalin into the bloodstream, where it travels to another location in the body to have its effect. An example of this would be when adrenalin secreted by the adrenal gland would travel through the blood stream to the heart where it would cause the heart to beat rapidly.

A good analogy for the water soluble neurotransmitter system is the marketplace. For example, a large store makes an order for a product. Let's use the example of t-shirts. A large t-shirt order is placed by WalMart. The factory goes to work and produces a large batch of t-shirts. These t-shirts are bundled into large bundles and placed in large trucks that drive a long way on the freeway to get to the WalMart store. And at the store, all the t-shirts are unloaded at once.

This is similar to the water soluble neurotransmitters that are produced in bulk far away from the synapse. The water soluble chemicals are packaged in large bundles(vesicles). These vesicles are like the trucks that carry the t-shirts far away to the store. These large vesicles fill with the neurotransmitters and carry the neurotransmitters far away to the synapse, where they are unloaded all at once.

To summarize: the water soluble ante grade neurotransmitters are produced at a separate location from the synapse, travel down the neuron to the synapse, and release a large amount of neurotransmitter each time they are released. The retrograde or backward signaling of the endocannabinoid system is much different (Fig 10,11). The endocannabinoid neurotransmitter is fat soluble. Because of the characteristics of fat soluble chemicals, endocannabinoid neurotransmitters cannot travel through the body and have a remote effect. This means that the lipid soluble endocannabinoid neurotransmitter is produced locally. Indeed, we find the fat-soluble endocannabinoid molecules are produced from the lipid membrane of the posterior synapse, right out of the cell wall. These molecules travel the short distance backwards across the cleft to attach to its own unique G receptor. When the lipid soluble neurotransmitter occupies the receptor, the receptor then causes a chemical reaction that shuts off the release of water-soluble neurotransmitters into the pre-synaptic cleft. This means the postsynaptic neuron can literally shut off the stimulation coming from the presynaptic neurons. This causes incoming stimuli to the postsynaptic neuron to be decreased. The locally produced fat soluble reverse neurotransmitters shut off the oncoming water soluble neurotransmitters, stopping them from working. This is why endocannabinoids are able to dampen or decrease stimuli in the nervous system. Cannabinoids have been called the "dimmer" switch for the nervous system. Another way to look at cannabinoids is that they "veto" the release of the water soluble ante grade neurotransmitters, nullifying their signal. They act as a vast network of locally active lipid neurotransmitters that is a buffer to the water soluble neurotransmitters throughout the body.

As the large vesicles release (dump) their water soluble chemicals into the synaptic cleft, the concentration of the water soluble neurotransmitters can get too high and injure the neuron. It is at that time fat soluble "keys" are made right out of the cell wall of the posterior synapse. These unique fat soluble keys go backwards to the presynaptic neuron. They fit into the CB receptor protein in the presynaptic neuron and cause a chemical reaction that shuts off the release of the water soluble neurotransmitter. So the endocannabinoid system acts like a fat soluble buffer that modifies the water soluble release. It acts like a "fat suit' that coats the nervous system to make a buffer system that "dims" the action of the water soluble neurotransmitters when they become too strong. It vetoes the water soluble neurotransmitters.

Cannabinoid receptors are the most frequently found receptors in the Nervous system, making up more than two-thirds of all neuroreceptors in the Nervous system.

Further research showed that endocannabinoids are two thirds of the G receptors in the central nervous system.[10] This means that the majority of receptors in the central nervous system are retrograde messengers. This means that the post synaptic receiving neuron can reach backwards and modify the function of the incoming presynaptic neuron. In this way the receiving neuron can alter the message it is receiving. This message is usually used to "turn down or decrease" the stimuli the postsynaptic neuron feels. This is the cannabinoid "dimmer switch" for the central nervous system. This decreases neurotransmitter signal and cools down the postsynaptic nerve. Before this knowledge of cannabinoids, all neurotransmitters were thought to proceed in one direction only, ante grade. To sum up the present day knowledge we can say that cannabis is a fat soluble reverse neurotransmitter with a unique G receptor.

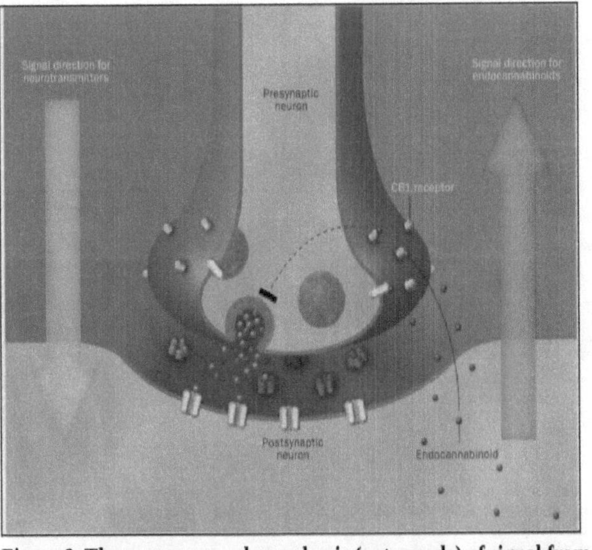

Figure 9 The green arrow shows classic (ante grade) of signal from the presynaptic neuron to postsynaptic neuron. The orange arrow shows the reverse (retrograde) direction of the endocannabinoid signal, from the postsynaptic neuron to the presynaptic neuron.